# The Insomniacs Guide to Sleep

# Copyright



First Printing: 2019

ISBN: 9781687141781

Kindle Publishing

79 Shelthorpe Avenue
Loughborough
Leicestershire
LE11 2ND

# Disclaimer

The opinions and suggestions expressed in this book are solely my own.
The reader or listener takes full responsibility when undertaking any of the suggestions expressed throughout this book.
This book is purely for entertainment purposes and not to be taken as medical or factual advice.

# Table of contents

# Introduction:

Okay so here goes. Imagine a Psychologically unhinged person recommending the right medication for you after years of there own experiences and taking them. well, that's just how this book started. Around the age of 14 I discovered I had serious sleeping issues to the point I was prescribed sleeping tablets it was kind of unheard back then for my age group. I substituted with many other things over the years, but I would still find myself sometimes awake for weeks in a row and back on medications to get me back into a sleep pattern that I never really had in the first place.

I can feed you all the usual crap.

Cut out the Caffeine, eat a light meal for supper free from red meats and fish.

Try turkey-based evening meals with bananas as a snack. Don't drink carbonated beverages or sugar-based fruit juices but you've probably tried everything already from Acupuncture to Hypnosis just to try and get an ounce of shut-eye.

My First Advice...Stop Trying. that's it give up trying to sleep.

Embrace your insomnia,

# Chapter 1
# The Bedroom

So, it's a simple term right Bedroom? Yet we turn this space into the most stressful activity centre in the whole house. You name it we create it.
Sex sanctuary
Home office
Pets paradise
Children's play haven
Library
It's a bedroom god damn it a bed in a room that's what it should be about when you're trying to sleep. Get a storage bed put everything underneath it not your pets obviously, but laptops, televisions, separate your spaces do not have any screens around your bedroom when you are sleeping.
Nowadays Alexa or Siri can play us a Lullaby, but you can hide them away from view and listen to ambient sounds or binaural beats depending on your preference.
I quite like heavy rain jeez I once had a picture with sound on the wall it was a cool thing back then, but it did the opposite of helping you sleep it was downright weird and creaked a lot. Thank god

Technology has moved on so you can listen to realistic sounds of nature Nowadays.
I remember my first water feature trying to balance the Feng shui in my first place.
Every morning it would wake me up gurgling, the last mouthful of water as the last drop dripped onto my very new carpet it didn't last long, to say the least.
That was all about creating peace and harmony within my home yet again I neglected to apply the same techniques to my sleeping area.
I'm 41 now and only this year have I finally bought a bed that I find 100% comfortable.
We buy beds for our budgets yet spent ridiculous amounts of money on items of less importance.
just for example. Bed £129, Xbox £329.
Seriously I cannot stress this enough get the best bed you've ever had.
A nice couch or tv will not fix your bad back, health problems or insomnia, but a good bed and mattress will.
Once you have the basic's you can start creating your world of Zen.
Sex and insomnia! The amount of times I've heard people say good sex gives you better sleep. Yes, after a marathon sex session or explosive orgasm you will sleep, but try and keep that up night after night with a job and a family or even just yourselves eventually you'll be exhausted and not in a good way. Beds are not as resilient as people think.
Dreams didn't have 8 years of sex acrobatics in mind with its replacement figure. A year of the honeymoon period on a cheap bed and whoops bad back alert. I'm not saying don't do it. Just respect your bed and protect it accordingly get mattress toppers and keep your mattress nice and firm for back support. Prevention is better than cure remember!
So Anyway, where was I yes, your bed.
Get a Good one and Look after it with your life and it will look after your back. you back you know what I mean.

My boy has no trouble sleeping on his back in My bed little bugger!!

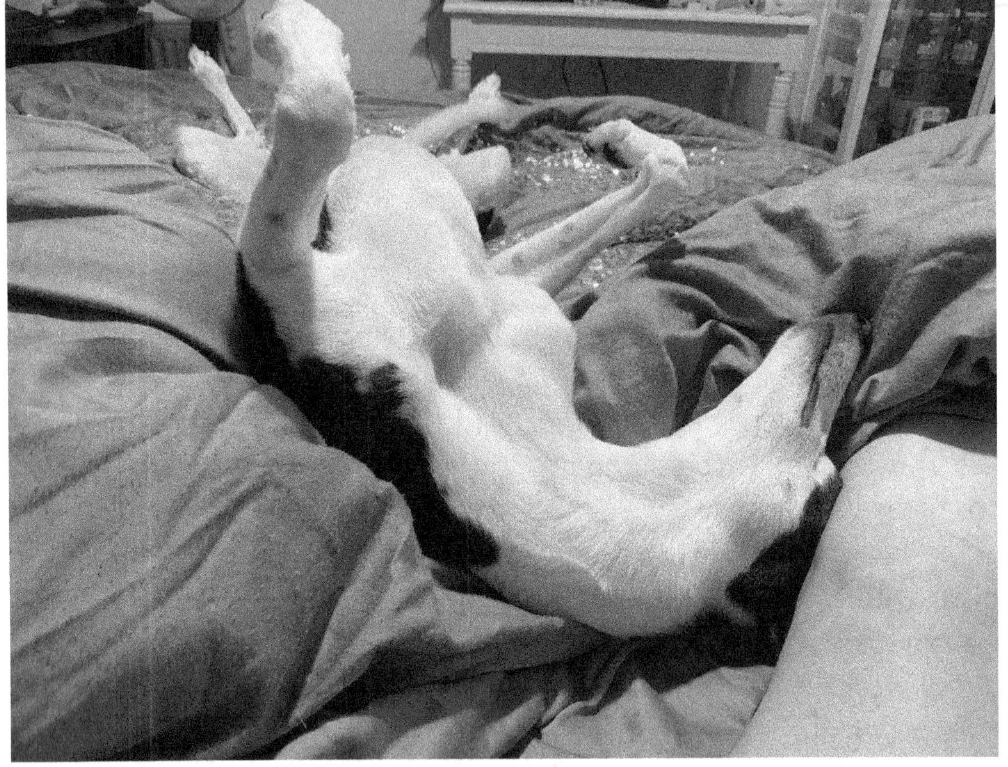

# Chapter 2
## Advice, guidance? not on your nelly

Do something creative. write a book even.
Sleep with your animals, dogs' cats, etc. let them snooze on your bed.
Yes, they fart, snore leave hairs, but humans leave a mess!
To the dust in our houses made from hair, nails, and skin too.
I apologize to the weak-stomached of our world but it's just science.
If you haven't got a pet get a Teddy.
yes, grown adults can get Teddy's.
The point I'm trying to make is creating a nurturing safe and secure environment for yourself.
Get Blackout blinds... if you don't like the dark use low wattage fairy lights to give you a little light but not that bright, they will disturb you.
Take Water to bed sometimes we all need a sip or two.
Buy comfortable nightclothes.
A lot of people choose seductive wear over comfort but let's face it if you are not sleeping you are not feeling at your best anyway. Rest and recharge before you ramp up the ramrod.
you'll both feel the benefit.
Did I say remove pets before engaging in any activity?
Sometimes we need a hot drink, get up and get one. Caffeine-free though of course.
Never check the time. Ever!! It is a guaranteed curse to keep you awake night after night.

# Chapter 3
# Just for fun

Have you ever wondered what nightwalkers do?
Don't!! if you can't handle horror movies. If your intrigued read on.

They just walk around at night that's it!! Pray to the moon may be cast a few spells by the light of the moon. Recharge their crystals there are probably fewer evil goings-on than in the daylight hours. Sometimes the dark can be our friend.

The Stars come out at night, the sky is filled with a map of the universe with amazing constellations as old as time itself if we all slept under a blanket of the sky with no distractions, beeps, screen lights
Or devices on stand-by wed sleep a little sounder.

Sometimes the sound of an oscillating fan in the corner of a room can bring comfort to some.
Lavender drops on a pillow a hot bath before bed can all be a simple solution even camomile tea helps some drift off to cloudphoria. All I say is don't give yourself such a hard time.

Sometimes your Brain is simply saying I've still got work stuff out so I can't shut off yet.
 So, distract the impeccable child. you're in charge it's your brain.
Give it something too good to refuse. I'm my case I can watch a

certain cartoon and then that's all I can think about so I'm lying in bed with a stupid smile on my face but hey it works!

Laughter is the best medicine it's not a new phenomenon
Try it.
Smiling does something to your brain, told you I'm nuts but hey lying in bed smiling your head off at night will help you sleep because sooner or later you'll be laughing at yourself for looking like a smiling weirdo that much you will get face ache from it. Don't knock it till you've tried it. If you start laughing and looking like a crazy person just go with it. let it out.
Then take a deep breath and enjoy the euphoric feeling afterwards.
Happy Sleeping Mad Hatters
We all go a little crazy Sometimes.

# Chapter 4

# Now for the serious stuff

So, I 've had a little joke and if you did embrace your insomnia and clear your room, you're really on the right road to actually cure yourself.

The fact I said accept your insomnia is it is all in our minds literally, yet it seeps into everyday life and causes us to underperform at work, get angry with people put on weight and causes depression. This can lead to a whole heap of mental health issues.

If we drive were putting other people as well as ourselves at risk driving tired. Sleep is the foundation of life and physical health.

Stop telling yourself you cannot sleep it's a negative affirmation your brain is hearing every time you say it. Instead tell yourself you can sleep you were born being able to sleep you slept like a baby, child and even as a teenager. You might have only just started being wakeful at night and you're in your 20's. Age is irrelevant but the amount of sleep you actually need is the important factor.

But do not get yourself worked up if you don't sleep for that long I still believe in quality over quantity
If you want to analyse your sleep get yourself a Fitbit and analyse it yourself, you could be getting more than you think but it's not the quality you require. The Fitbit Versa will tell you your waking periods as well as restlessness, just get one second-hand from E-bay most people buy these things brand new and never really use them normally around January when they join a gym for one month and then quit. I hold my hands up there as I have done the same with a gym pass many times.

Christmas goodies followed by the new year resolutions I now just go with the flow probably why I am a size 16 but what the heck I am happier than I have ever been.

It could do with the sleep I am getting nowadays.

# Chapter 5

# The bedtime routine

Do not go to bed telling yourself you can't sleep or won't sleep.
Eliminate all outside disturbances.
If you find yourself thinking about stuff tell yourself not to think.
Lie flat on your back, arms down by your side and tighten everything from your eyes, facial muscles hands, to your toes count to ten slowly and let go.
Does these ten times and feel your muscles relax more each time until you have fully let your whole body go floppy including your eye muscles, mouth muscles and fingertips.
Now concentrate on your breathing.
Breath in slowly, feel your chest moving and breath out.
Do these ten times always keep your eyes closed and body relaxed.

If any of you are parents and your little ones have unfortunately been a fan or still is a fan of in the night garden, you will understand what I mean but imagine your iggle wiggle in his little boat drifting out to sea on a boat. Or just be yourself in a little boat drifting on a calm see in a blanket of stars sleeping as you drift effortlessly along the calm sea or lake. Still breathing deeply and slowly in and out.

Imagine this until you feel relaxed.

If you're not a lover of the sea but love nature. Be the relaxed person on a hammock swinging gently in the tree's peaceful and tranquil with maybe the sounds that soothe you like a babbling brook.

Maybe you like to sleep by a cosy fire in a wooden cottage laid out on the most luxurious rug with the person of your dreams.

The fact is we can create our nurturing environment in our minds and every night we can go back and visit in the world of restful sleep.

Imagine sleep like a book you are reading so your excited to know what's going to happen next and you will love going to bed and creating your sleeping novel.

Find out what comforts you and build on that.
Create your space of sleep physically and mentally.

Let me know how you get on

Drop me a message at

https://www.becksterboo.co.uk/

# Chapter 6

# Eating at night

In my earlier chapters, I joked about eating the right foods
But certain foods have substances in them that help you sleep.

Bananas:
 help you sleep because they contain magnesium and potassium
both of which are very good for relaxing the muscles.
As well as containing the amino acid L-tryptophan which converts in
the brain to a substance that helps us sleep better.

Turkey:
 Again, turkey contains tryptophan's but as a good source of protein
will make you feel full. Ever wondered why everyone falls asleep
after dinner at Christmas. That's the reason why.

Almonds:
 Almonds contain both magnesium and tryptophan's so a double
whammy here just like bananas to relax those muscles and produce
melatonin which naturally occurs in the brain for sleep.

Oats:

Have you ever tried eating porridge before bed, lacing it with sugar and syrup will have the opposite effect but top it with bananas and crushed almonds and you will have cracked the Bowl of sleep porridge.

Honey:

If you prefer something sweeter on your porridge, then the good news is honey will also help produce melatonin that's why the age-old warm milk and honey gets used a lot.

# Chapter 7

## Foods to avoid

These foods may seem obvious to some, but others seem to think they have the opposite effect,

Alcohol
Alcohol might make you pass out, but it gives you the worst type of sleep if you suffer from not sleeping avoid alcohol at night like the plague.

Cheese;
A lot of us love a bit of cheese especially with biscuits at night but it can have the opposite effect as cheese contains something that makes your brain more alert ever wondered why people mention having strange dreams after cheese?

Caffeine
Anything that contains caffeine will keep you awake and not help you sleep at all.

Spicy foods;

Having a vindaloo might be tempting after a few beers but you are fighting a losing battle. For one, you won't fall into a deep sleep and to top it all off you will probably suffer horrendous heartburn as a side effect.

High sugar and fatty foods;

We all do it munch on sweets and chocolates watching our favourite series before we go to bed but we are heading for a sugar crash and fatty food especially yet again lead to heartburn.

# Chapter 8

# Things to try

Some of us are terrified of strenuous exercise I know I am.
The thing is exercise does help not the stuck in the doors with fake lighting type but the exposure to natural sunshine type.

Our bodies produce melatonin when it is dark and produce less when its light that's why backlit devices in the dark are having the opposite effect on our bodies.
Eliminate screens 2 hours before bed. Keep your room as dark as possible.
Never watch TV in bed then expect to fall asleep straight after it just will not happen unless your body is exhausted but again the quality of sleep is not the best when your body shuts down.

I love my DVDs but keep them for the weekends.

Having a lie in feels great but if you get up at 12 pm on a Sunday you are not going to sleep well Sunday night before work on a Monday.

Keep your bedtime routine consistent and don't try and marathon sleep at weekends. Instead get out and get some fresh air, have a brisk walk.

If you find you have children that don't sleep take them out do something fun and engaging that uses physical and mental abilities. Never keep them up late hoping they will sleep better or longer that will overstimulate them and you're asking for a whole heap of mental health problems to follow.

Sleep is one of the most important human needs so do everything you can to make sure you can get some.
Get the basics right and you won't even have to try, it will just happen naturally, and you'll wonder why it wasn't so simple before.

# Resources

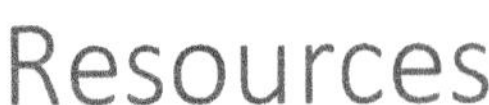

https://www.helpguide.org/home-pages/sleep.htm


https://www.helpguide.org/articles/sleep/sleep-needs-get-the-sleep-you-need.htm


https://www.msn.com/en-ph/health/mindandbody/the-military-technique-to-fall-asleep-in-two-minutes/ar-BBQjOxn

YouTube help to sleep videos


https://youtu.be/69o0P7s8GHE


https://youtu.be/63vw6fUVhBQ